HEALTH CARE AND FREEDOM

An American Dilemma

James Hill Parker
Long Island University, Brooklyn, N.Y.

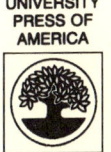

UNIVERSITY
PRESS OF
AMERICA

Lanham • New York • London

Copyright © 1994 by
University Press of America®, Inc.
4720 Boston Way
Lanham, Maryland 20706

3 Henrietta Street
London WC2E 8LU England

Library of Congress Cataloging-in-Publication Data
Parker, James Hill.
Health care and freedom : an American dilemma /
by James Hill Parker.
p.   cm.
Includes index.
1. Huntington's chorea—Patients—Nursing home care—New Jersey.
2. Social medicine—United States. 3. Medical care—United States.
I. Title.
RC394.H85P37   1993   362.1—dc20   93–31127 CIP

ISBN 0–8191–9302–X (cloth : alk. paper)
ISBN 0–8191–9303–8 (pbk. : alk. paper)

 The paper used in this publication meets the minimum requirements of
American National Standard for Information Sciences—Permanence
of Paper for Printed Library Materials, ANSI Z39.48–1984.

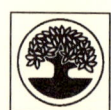

Good people can
overcome a bad system

And good systems can
prevail over bad people

But bad people in a bad system
points the way to catastrophe.

However, good people in a good
system can work miracles.

Lecture notes,
1977
by Author

Dedicated
to

My wife, Alice,

who, like the rest of us,
must suffer through disease and death.

also

My sister-in-law,
Jane W. Parker,

who, having known this tragedy three times,
helped the author understand
that beyond all the confusion
was a wholeness which was spiritual in nature
and expressed in caring and love.

and

My daughter, Lisa,

who was an immense help throughout
the entire process.

Acknowledgements

The dedication page indicates the most important persons in this study. However, others have contributed as well, such as my son James and my son in law John. The scattering of social workers, nurses and others who helped along the process are the good people in a bad health system.

The Huntington's Disease Society of New Jersey also deserves credit in helping along the process, especially Rhoda Grossman and Alice Lazzarini. Other people, too numerous to mention, contributed in their own way, including churches, friends and relatives.

The research time and assistance given by Long Island University and my colleagues is also greatly appreciated.

Also, the State of New Jersey deserves great credit for funding and establishing the health care "experiment" described at the end of the book.

Finally, my daughter Lisa, who, through her persistence, was instrumental in getting her mother placed in a caring environment.

TABLE OF CONTENTS

INTRODUCTION

It is not often that a sociologist can comment on an intense personal experience through the use of his or her own Sociological imagination and practice.

In this case, the sociology of health and bureaucracy came to the fore as a personal experience and participant observation of the most intense kind.

Because of the personal emotional involvement here, it is all the more crucial that objectivity of some kind be maintained. To secure this end, the use of four other observers has been employed, to check on the accuracy, indeed the essential validity of such an endeavor. The observers consist of the patient, another sociologist, and two relatives. To this end, we have found a large amount of agreement on the following events and their versions and interpretations. Needless to say, this essential agreement does not constitute proof, for the agreement was based on ongoing construction of reality through common terms and common logics. In other words the participant observers' conclusions were based on prior world views and all it suggests. Moreover, the observers arrived at consensus through interaction, thus it was an interactionally constructed consensus painfully put together through the dubious means of talking.

Nevertheless, we shall depend on this socially arrived at reality to make some sense out of the events and interpretations to follow for there appears to be no other way to do it.

It often happens that we learn more from our adversaries than our friends. This appears to be the case here. We have taken serious account of the versions of our bureaucratic and other adversaries as well as so-called neutral observers. As we know, there are no neutral observers for they all have their stories based as they are upon other world views, vocabularies and vested moral and other interests.

The best we can do in this or any other case is to construct a composite reality from a variety of viewpoints based as they are, upon each person's closely held, and heavily guarded personal and social identities.

The fact that there are larger blocks of unknowables on the part of everyone concerned makes this endeavor even more perilous. The further fact that secrecy is the mainstay of all organizations and persons in them compounds the difficulty of knowing even more.

With these considerations in mind, we shall, nevertheless, proceed in the name of science, intuition and experience to construct a version of one case of individuals caught in a maze of medical, organizational and indeed, community structures and procedures.

This one case we feel is not unusual, but rather a paradigm of a much larger problem of citizens caught in similar no-win situations in modern societies. It is also a paradigm, we think, of why larger structures in a mass society do not work and indeed cause problems of their own at the macro-level.

I. THE PROBLEM OF HEALTH CARE

It seems the best place to begin a story of this kind is at the beginning, or at least what we choose to call the beginning.

On two separate occasions, my wife was burned by lighting herself on fire through careless use of smoking materials. Ordinarily this should not be a great problem. However, in her case, she had been stricken over a period of years with Huntington's Disease. Huntington's Disease is an inherited neuro-physical disease, where brain cells die or become nonfunctional after a period of time. The usual onset is at about 40 years of age. Certain areas of the brain are affected, which results in a continuing loss of motor control. Also, it appears that in some cases judgement and thinking and emotional centers are affected. The progress of the disease averages 15 years, resulting in death, often from lack of ability to eat or from pneumonia caused by inhaled food particles. This condition resulted in carelessness in behavior in general and a lack of physical coordination. Thus what was a careless accident with matches and cigarettes began on two different occasions with hospital stays of some length, and after the second accident, admission to a so-called nursing home.

The story to follow is the story of medical and social service mismanagement. What could have been a smooth transition between hospital and nursing home became a horror story of sorts. Even in the best of situations transferring a loved one into a nursing home is usually traumatic for relatives. Often, according to one social worker's version, relatives feel guilt, sorrow and confusion, and experience sort of a roller coaster of emotions and ideational shifts, often in rapid succession, and usually for a long period of time (in some cases forever).

Not only is a social arrangement - the family - broken up, but in many cases a lifetime of relationships that now become, for all practical purposes, defunct.   In short, relatives experience a great loss, oddly enough, often greater than the loss through death.

There is a certain finality about death.

There is no such finality with lingering illnesses - which must be dealt with day after day, week after week, hour after hour.

Seeing a lingering illness turned into a separation of a loved one into a nursing home or facility can be much worse. Having limited access to such a facility, as we will discuss here, is even worse - intolerable. To see the loved one in virtual prison - a prisoner of the nursing home - is to a sensitive person probably the worst case scenario.

Some people admittedly will merely cut off all contacts with the loved one and treat them for practical purposes dead. This is often the case.

However, others, such as myself refuse to or cannot do this. Their loved one is _alive, aware,_ and in _need_ - in a hostile or at best in a non-caring world.

Patients also vary in their reaction to confinement.

The ones who are _aware_ suffer most. In their case, they retreat eventually into a small world - or according to another social worker's version, they _settle in._

The truth is many _aware_ persons _do not_ settle in. For that matter, as we will discuss later, they don't settle for any of it. Some become hostile, some seethe in resentment and bitterness and others form small cliques to reenact the social world from which they came with concerns about status, rights, fights and territory.

Among the aware, visits from anyone become critically important if for no other reason than it gives them status and position, or the visits are a symbol that they are still part of that critical unit, the family, or in some cases, the church or friendship groups from the outside.

Some families who visit come to be seen as hostile intruders by the nursing home personnel, especially family members who criticize or make demands on the system. We shall discuss more of this later, having had that particular experience of being labeled a troublemaker or a potential threat to the nursing home, doctors, hospital and social service agencies.

And as we shall see later, each organization involved with caring for the patient sees their first problem as protecting themselves from the public, higher authority and damaging complaints.

Aside from the hidden agendas of organizations involved, there are also hidden agendas of the individuals in the organizations. First among these is _careerism._ The career overwhelms, in most cases, the problems of the patients, their relatives and even their own organizations. We shall give examples of this throughout.

Also, each individual in health care or other organizations brings their own personal problems, opinions and belief systems to their work.

In many cases, health professionals have problems of overwork and underpay along with political hassles with other workers in the same or different organizations. Personality quirks are also brought to the job from garden variety problems and behaviors to drug addiction and in a few cases outright psychopathic behavior. To say the least, the patient in any setting does not benefit from these things.

Abuse of patients, physical and psychological, results often from so-called health professionals' personal and organizational problems.

There is much to be said for sympathizing with these health professionals. They are after all victims of larger systems, namely and especially national health policy and its attendant pressures. This high level policy, such as cuts in funds, dribbles down to create alienated health care workers, from the alienation of high paid physicians to alienation of very low paid nurses and their even lower paid assistants such as L.P.N.'s, janitors and cooks.

This alienation at all levels eventually impinges upon millions of patients, especially Medicaid patients - they become in the eyes of health workers a nuisance. The patient becomes the enemy. The "law suit" becomes the threat, and the family or the patients themselves become the instrument of pain and disaster even for physicians.

So the problem herein discussed, from top to bottom, is probably in part a problem of national health policy, but at lower levels - a disdain and even hatred for the sick and infirmed. For indeed Social Darwinism is still with us at all levels. That is, a version of blaming the victim is part of the American dream and blaming the victim is a logical antidote for explaining the American nightmare, contradiction to this dream. The poor, the sick, must be explained away. What better way of explaining them away than the belief that people get what they deserve.

There are of course attacks against the notion of the American dream. This is nowhere more evident than the attacks against the health care system or non-system. It is becoming increasingly evident that extremely sophisticated American medical technology is not being delivcred evenly, and this is especially evident among the most helpless members of our society: the very young, the very old, and the very poor.

Perhaps the only reason the medical part of the dream is being questioned is because the middle and even the upper middle class is also being affected.

So it is especially appropriate that this critique focuses on an upper middle class family.

In brief, catastrophic illness can affect any family to the point of tragedy, except perhaps for the upper 10% or 15% of the income distribution.

In short, catastrophic illness affects, or can affect, so many people that it has become a major political issue.

Oddly enough as the length of life increases, the possibility of catastrophic, long-term illness increases. It is a case of success breeding more problems.

In any case, we find that social policies and problems at the state or national or international level have a direct impact on individuals. Individuals unfortunately do not always see their problems as widely shared and a reflection of larger societal problems and as a result blame themselves or have some vague idea that the society is wrong or evil.

Paradoxically, individual problems such as a general preoccupation with death and disease generate problems that larger structures must try to address. Whether the larger structures be religious, political, scientific or any other institution, there is always the possibility that the larger structure cannot cope with it or comes up with faulty solutions. So, there is a certain circularity to problems from top to bottom, and bottom to top, meeting somewhere in the middle as in organizations. This is certainly true of medical problems in our culture.

This organizational range where individual and societal problems and solutions meet can be well documented in the field of medicine, illness and death.

The nursing home is only one of these organizational types. However, it is where the critical failures and problems at all levels often meet. Nursing homes pick up where every other medical or health care program fails. It is in a sense a trash heap of failures of other structures or organizations.

As we have mentioned, the catastrophic illnesses and the hordes of victims are the endpoint in many cases of successful, medical and societal interventions - by extending life function to the point where we no longer are sure who is legally dead and legally alive.

We should be aware that, for example, third world countries have very few nursing homes because they have very poor health care, so die young for the most part.

Other structures in the middle range in the health care industry range widely - including not only the usual hospital, doctor, dentist list but also include a wide variety of industries and things as diverse as: occupations, drug stores, mortuaries, self-help groups, churches, insurance companies, medical supply companies and medical waste companies.

II. THE CASE STUDY AND THE SCAMS

The hospital was the best place - where the accident was treated, but again the intervention of well (?) meaning officials, social workers and others caused all hell for everybody concerned.

The accident was one common to many Huntington's Disease patients who smoke, according to affected families and professionals who deal with disease.

This accident was the setting on fire of my wife's (nylon) blouse by herself in another room. She was forever dropping lighted cigarettes on herself, furniture and carpeting. She was badly burned and spent six weeks in the hospital.

The social workers did their job upon release from the hospital of my wife. Because of insurance guidelines, she had to be out. She wanted to go home as always, and we knew this catastrophe could not happen again.

The social worker "placed" her in a nursing home in central New Jersey. It was a prison and it smelled of rotting flesh and garbage and my wife kept to herself. The prisoners <u>knew</u> they were in prison, and those who could, formed their own social world, imitating the real (?) one or ones they had come from. One patient said initially, "Do not say anything ... it will get you in trouble."

She was right. As I began to ask questions, answers appeared, but resulted in the police being called because of an altercation with a nurse (over a cup of coffee).

The place was being closed down by the state at the time. Everyone was distraught.

Perhaps as a reward (?) for my efforts, she (my wife) now deteriorated, was placed in a second "home".

Physically, it was a bit superior but again a prison run by a Warden.

Deciding not to be a "troublemaker," I proceeded as usual and as recommended (by the experts of various sorts) to pay attention to my wife's care and to be very nice.

The Incident

I mentioned to a nurse's aide that the dayroom television was for the patients, not the staff, and that they (the nurses' aides) were blocking it and controlling it.

Since histories follow Medicaid records, I had obviously been recorded formally or informally as a troublemaker and somebody to watch.

The owner/director had me set up thereafter.

This is not paranoia. Soon after the TV incident, we came at night to visit, met at the door by a raging - screaming nurse (who had been fired from four jobs in five months), accusing us without provocation of being troublemakers. (We had not said a word.)

The next day, the owner was called, the story being given, and she said she would check into it. In an hour she returned the call (protecting herself) saying in effect, "You caused problems. You are a troublemaker." The nurse wrote down a very different story. "If you do this again," (me, my daughter and son-in-law were all there, by the way), "I shall call the police," the director said.

A few hours later the director called again and said she wanted to meet with me. I said okay. I took my daughter as a witness. It was not very civil, but well constructed. The director of nursing was her witness as it were, and we all sat down. The owner was not used to serious confrontation. Anyway, the proceedings proceeded with a not too veiled threat that with the least provocation, the police would be called (for what?) and besides we didn't need to be there all the time.

Obviously, this system was operational. The Medicaid troublemaker record was probably there and we all felt trapped. A series of events that followed which I shall describe only briefly that consisted of: "accidents" happening to my wife, threats that she would be put in a mental hospital, continuous complaints on the director's part about my wife's Bad Behavior or being a problem. Also, when the notary public showed up there to sign some papers for me, he was told to leave.

Yes, we were being harassed in a major way.

When my wife said she had been beaten on a number of occasions, this was the last straw.

[THIS IS A NATIONAL SCENARIO
AND A BIG PROBLEM
FOR
20-30 MILLION PATIENTS AND FAMILIES]

Keeping in mind throughout all of this, that organizations everywhere protect first and foremost themselves, their careers and at the expense of those they are supposed to serve.

In any case, we got no satisfaction from anybody at the "home," except a "turncoat" nurse (who believed in truth) who was soon fired.

A letter was written to the state health agencies (with copies to relevant others of course) to ask for an investigation. (Yes, this is being a "TROUBLEMAKER".)

They, the state agencies, Ombudsmen, etc., of course found nothing, but did approve her transfer.

State of New Jersey

DEPARTMENT OF HUMAN SERVICES
DIVISION OF MEDICAL ASSISTANCE AND HEALTH SERVICES

LOCAL AREA OFFICE

4/18/90

Dr. James H. Parker

--------, NJ -----

                Re: Alice Parker
                        1320-009205-01

Dear Dr. Parker:

      This is in response to your complaint against -----
Nursing Home regarding your wife.

      Your allegations have been investigated by my staff and they could not be substantiated. As you stated in your letter, the Department of Health has agreed to investigate separately.

      Your request for the transfer of your wife to another facility has been approved by separate letter.

                        Sincerely yours,

                        -----, Director
                        ----- MDO

The system had worked for those in the system.   (Why am I not surprised?)

Earlier, we had written to the county Medicaid office, with copies to the State of New Jersey and the social worker from the Huntington's Disease Association:

```
                                  ------------------
                                  --------, N.J. -----

                                  April 5, 1990



Medicaid Office
-------------
------, New Jersey -----

        Re:   State of New Jersey
              --------------, M.S.W.
              Huntington's Disease Association, N.J.

Dear ------------:

        I have been referred to you by -------------- of the
Huntington's Disease Association concerning the transfer of
Alice Parker to another nursing home facility.  Alice
Parker, who is my wife, is currently living at the -------
Nursing home in ------, New Jersey.

        The reasons I am requesting a transfer are many.  The
first and foremost of my concerns is that she is being
physically abused by a nurse's aide.  I have received this
information from my wife.  The nurse's aide abuses my wife
on the weekends - such as hitting her in the face.

        I have already contacted the State Department of
Health.  They have agreed to investigate my wife's
complaints against the nurse's aide.  I am fearful this
situation could become progressively worse.  Please
consider her transfer to a more caring environment.

                              Sincerely,


                              Dr. James H. Parker
```

III. THE EXPERIMENT IN FREEDOM AND DIGNITY

Enter the Huntington's Association. At last a solution appeared because only systems can beat or fight systems.

The Huntington's Disease Association was <u>a system with big connections.</u>

It now came into play, finally after much prodding. My daughter called a social worker who suggested she (my wife) be examined at the University Hospital where the Huntington's research unit was located in an adjoining county.

The appointment was made, my wife transported, and at which time she was asked if she had been beaten.

She said, "Yes."

Again asked, she said, "Yes."

That was enough for ---------, social worker for the Association.

People hate to hear about helpless people getting beaten. She, my wife, fortunately was soon shifted to a newly-founded and funded nursing complex under the auspices of the Association and the state which begins another story.

Suffice it to say, we had now entered a better system, but again a system (a powerful system) with its own agenda, its own careers at stake, and again protecting itself, albeit more beneficently than many other systems.

An analysis of the Huntington's unit <u>system</u> will constitute the bulk of the rest of this book.

By this time (1990) I had probably gained a reputation which I was determined <u>not</u> to reinforce in this new, beneficent and magnificent setting.

Initially, of course, I was merely grateful - like the "Grateful Dead." Yes, truly I was. I was amazed at this place. It cost between $50,000 and $100,000 a year per patient (which I did not have to pay because we had no resources, being impoverished by the medical costs). It was staffed with therapists; a social worker who ran "socio-emotional" groups each week, an occupational therapist, a speech therapist and a recreational therapist.

This was for only 15 patients, all with the same disease.

A truly remarkable step forward.

The research design basis of this operation, benign as it appeared to be, gradually became apparent. Again, I had stumbled into a fascinating world where an experiment was being conducted -as a model upon which other systems would be built with worldwide attention on its outcome - for it was to become, if successful, a model for handling other kinds of disease populations.

I shall not be cynical about what I had discovered using my own (medical sociology) methodologies for assessing and uncovering this intriguing experiment.

Unfortunately, as we shall see, one methodology (of the Huntington's Unit experiment) ran into and defended itself against another methodology (namely my own); seemingly unobtrusive participant observation measures of understanding this wonderful new world of dealing with the dying and later the relatives and finally the problems that plague all organizations.

The following could also be called research designs and methodology in potential collision.

At this point, the analysis becomes more of a problem of conducting research anywhere, even when you do not mean any harm except perhaps to a nonfunctional national health care problem which must be solved.

This place, I think, is the beginning of a solution or an attempt at it.

The problem, though, is that the problem is a structural-political problem at the national level. The current systems of National Health, i.e., insurance companies, health professional associations, the structure of wealth and power in America places enormous constraints on what experiment an organization can do.

Also, what this "experiment" can do is affected, as everywhere, by the problems that employees bring to their work, including crises in their own life.

The amazing thing is that health care, or any organization works at all. We have said the systemic requirements of all organizations create their own problems.

Some of the problems created by organizations as they grow are the following:

1. The over-creation of bureaucracy and specialties which are created by the bureaucracy.
2. The Iron Law of Oligarchy, where powers move to the top of the organization.
3. The routinization of charisma, where a once creative set of ideas comes to be set in stone, even reversing the original charismatic goals.
4. The tendencies of organizations to grow beyond their necessary scope.
5. The tendency of organizations to become self protective, again perverting the original goals.
6. The emergence of informal organization which may undermine the formal structure.
7. The tendency of professional groups, especially in a post-industrial society, to develop their own power structures and fight with each other.

And finally:

8. The problem of <u>trained incapacity,</u> where people are overtrained to the degree that they can do little else than what they are trained for, and often not even that.

This particular analysis will perhaps be flawed by the personal-emotional involvement with a patient (my wife) being in the organization.

Thus, the eternal and practically insoluble problem of the purpose, the slant in interpretation of the investigator becomes a methodological problem. On the other hand, the (this) investigator must choose a level and type of analysis that is suitable to his conscious (and unconscious) purpose.

The question, at base, becomes what is the <u>purpose</u> of the methodology and what does the investigator purpose to do?

False starts, errors in judgment, and even being human, will even then cloud the social scientists' view of things.

At this point I would like to step back and rethink the project and whether or not to proceed further, and if so, reassess purpose, and the level of methodology that would be adequate to <u>that purpose</u>.

As I, or any other investigator, step back and look at what have been my purposes that I did and did not realize, it is clear that one purpose was to protect my wife.

IV. THE SOCIAL/ORGANIZATIONAL MODEL

There remains a further problem to be solved regarding purpose; that is, the purpose of those studied (e.g., the organization). In this case we have a compounded problem, for as far as I can see the nursing home, "the experiment", is in search of its own methodology. Its purpose partly then is that it has no specific methodology other than a vague orientation toward giving as much freedom as possible to patients and providing the best care. Beyond that the "organization" is in search of a methodology itself. It began without method largely and is in the process of exploring, finding a methodology.

This explains a conversation with the unit social worker who works part time. It went like this (paraphrased):

What is the purpose of your socio-emotional group sessions with patients?

Now really ... well, we just talk about things. Well, of course, the patient group cannot handle much.

Do you deal with any particular subject?

No ... no ... ahh ...

What is your theoretical orientation?

What?

What theory do you use? Freudian, meta-Freudian?

Well, really not any ... I mean, just whatever seems appropriate ... I guess it's an eclectic approach.

Well, what purpose do you have in this group?

We just talk.

About what?

Everything.

How interesting; a purposeless group. We now give an example of relatives' "support group," which is roughly paraphrased here.

"What is our purpose here?" she had asked in the meeting.
Nobody seemed to know.
"Do you want some chocolate cake," she had said.
"Yes, thanks." I took one.
"Coffee?"
"Yes, please."
"Well, let's go around the room and introduce ourselves. I'm ..."
"I'm ..." "I'm ...", etc.

Silence.
Some waitress carries on about something, attempting to exercise a control strategy. Everybody looked uncomfortable. "What do you think we should do?" the social worker asked.
Silence and confusion, etc.
"Would you like to have a picnic?"
"Yes, yes, yes." - general agreement.
When she asked "...do you all want to bring food?"
"Yes ... yes ... yes...", etc.
One old guy does not seem to care... just the women who apparently relate to the concept of "picnic."
"We could also take a trip with the patients."
Bus rides seemed to ring a bell but didn't go anywhere. Anyway, there seemed to be no purpose at the end except that we had even avoided the questions.

Nevertheless, the idea of the <u>free association group</u> is interesting. Even the concept of purpose has seemed through her to be irrelevant ... or a constant search, possibly.

So we have an organization trying to find the purpose(s) within broad objectives.

So, we have the interesting prospect of trying to devise a method of studying a place that is trying to find some purposes, and is indeed partly the reason for its existence.

So, we have a most interesting problem. It, "the organization," does appear to have limits to this freedom; not many, but some very interesting limits and some general purposes. I insert an article on the nursing home experiment here:

A MODEL CARE FACILITY TAKES SHAPE[*]
By Michael K. McCormack, Ph.D.

The Samuel L. Baily Huntington's Disease Family Service Center was founded in 1978 through an alliance of several faculty and staff of the University of Medicine and Dentistry of New Jersey (UMDNJ) and a number of families from the New Jersey Chapter of the then National Huntington's Disease Association (NHDA).

The original mission was to identify a group of medical and allied health professionals who would provide comprehensive, multidisciplinary services including neurology. psychiatry, medical genetics and genetic counseling, social services and rehabilitative services to people with HD and their family members. This continues to be our mission some 15 years later.

In June of 1982, a New Jersey family contacted a state legislator to describe an unfortunate situation involving the quality of care received by her two young sons affected by HD. This initial contact prompted the legislator to introduce Joint Resolution 20 on January 30, 1984, which directed "the Commissioner of Health to study the feasibility of establishing a residential care facility for patients with Huntington's Disease."

[*]   Reprinted from *The Marker*, Spring 1993, Huntington's Disease Society of America.

This resolution was signed by the Governor in April 1985 and the feasibility study concluded a year later. In the interim, having heard of the needs of New Jersey HD families, a second receptive legislator introduced a long-term care bill (February 1986) which authorized the allocation of $150,000 to establish a demonstration HD unit in New Jersey.

An informal meeting between the Governor and representative of the New Jersey NHDA Chapter prompted the Governor to double the appropriation to $300,000 and to sign the bill if passed by the New Jersey Legislature. The bill was duly passed by both the Senate and the Assembly, and the Governor signed it into law in February 1988.

The legislation called for the development of a demonstration long-term facility which would care for 15 to 20 residents with Huntington's Disease.

Little did we know that it would take another two years to identify a care facility that would be interested in the challenge of developing a long-term residential unit for HD. Negotiations to develop the facility at the -------- Center in ---------, NJ, were complex and involved the following important elements:

- The organization of the Huntington's Disease Family Service Center of UMDNJ, which had expertise in dealing with the complex needs of people with HD and their families;
- Identification of sympathetic key legislators by HD family members;
- A feasibility study to document the needs of HD families and to support the development of a demonstration long-term care unit;
- A budget surplus in New Jersey in 1985;
- A state law which mandated the creation of the unit, incentive start-up funding from the Legislature and a pre-negotiated Medicaid reimbursement rate of $274 per day per bed for a comprehensive care program.

Clearly a major incentive for enticing a center to accept the challenge of developing this unit was the enhanced Medicaid reimbursement rate without which the unit might never have been developed.

Today, the unit serves 16 residents with Huntington's Disease and provides several program features:

- Routine and specialty medical and dental services;
- Nursing services provided by personnel dedicated specially to the HD unit;
- Individual and family counseling by dedicated staff social workers and psychologist;
- Individual nutritional assessment and programming;
- Rehabilitative services including speech, occupational, physical and recreational therapies;
- Extramural activities such as swimming therapy, concerts, and field trips to New Jersey shore recreational parks.

The progress of the unit continues to be monitored by a review committee which reports to the state Department of Health and includes membership from various agencies such as Medicaid, the Department of Health, UMDNJ and the New Jersey Chapter of HDSA. The unit is now in its third year of operation and meets about 25% of the total need for residential care for New Jersey's HD residents. The program director and staff continue to seek innovative methods to improve communication skills and enhance quality of life for the residents. Likewise, there continues to be a need for day care and respite care programs which is currently under investigation.

Maintenance of function through comprehensive care continues to be the major focus of New Jersey Huntington's Disease programs, and while our successes have been limited, our resolve to continue is unquestionable.

In other words - the rule is, that there are limits to freedom, "this experiment in freedom."

For apparently, they know the "freedom" cannot exist without limits.

They are right of course.

How fascinating methodologically.   How to study freedom, only general purpose, so far, without disturbing its delicate balance.   I had already stepped over the bounds by asking questions.

"What is the purpose or the methodological problem now?"

It seems, that I just unobtrusively watch with the purpose of seeing what happens to freedom ... in this place without disturbing the process.

Having just "studied" nursing homes as prisons ... I now run into one that is obsessed with the limits of freedom.   What an opportunity methodologically and in a variety of, now unknown, number of ways.   At least I have stumbled into a radical comparative study of opposites and emergence of new "forms" of "dealing with?" patients where nothingness is even okay ... among staff and patients ... The nothingness of allowing a process of "freedom" working itself toward "being."

V. EXPERIMENT IN FREEDOM - WHAT HAPPENED TO IT?

What has happened to freedom in this great experiment, in this new nursing home, is now unfolding.

They have grouped together 15 people with the <u>same</u> disease and have stumbled into some of the problems of freedom or natural living among patients.

For the most part it has been a great success. Patients are not <u>over-medicated</u>, they are not constrained, they have a variety of real life and other activities like picnics, group eating, therapy and various social activities. They (the patients) are encouraged to be, to express, to develop themselves. For example, patients are encouraged, <u>not forced</u>, to become involved in discussion groups, play groups, parties and speech therapy. Some patients decline. It is accepted, and to this extent it constitutes freedom of choice with an opportunity structure for group involvement.

By the nature of the disease patients occasionally <u>lose it</u>, physically and emotionally.

They are allowed to fall, they occasionally fight or argue, but in the interest of giving them freedom, <u>not</u> neglect, for they are supervised and encouraged and taught by dedicated social work specialists.

However, the limits of freedom are gradually being approached such as the falling down and fighting that sometimes occurs. But to my knowledge, the patients <u>like this</u> freedom. The limits to freedom may well be the ability of the various levels of caretakers to tolerate this freedom. At the middle level (social workers and nurses) this does not seem to be critical yet. However, the lower level (nurses' aides) very occasionally lapse into apathy or authoritarianism. This is not to criticize them for they are really up against a control problem. The aides are low level and have a tough job. Some perform heroically, others do not.

The important thing here, though, is that most patients apparently like freedom, caring and structured activities. From my observation, some don't, however, want to attend things like psycho-social discussion groups. But then, they don't have to. If they want structure or structured groups, they can have it. If they don't want it, they don't have to participate. If we, outside the institution, could have that kind of freedom, we would be joyful indeed.

This program is indeed a model of nursing homes and other care of the institutionalized that works at least up to now. This freedom and privacy is indeed so protected that the intrusion by the investigation was blocked in a nice way. This was, and is, an experiment and the experiment was not to be intruded upon by an outside investigator or intruder.

Beyond cynicism, about protection of careers, and in the case of the doctors, reputations being part of it, the desire to run the course of the experiment for the benefit of the patients was paramount.

Yes, the patients are being experimented with, but for a noble purpose. I think namely to create or evolve a new model for caring for seriously impaired patients, but patients being seen as persons for the most part.

Beyond this, the cost of the experiment probably does not exceed the cost in corruption and malappropriation of Medicaid and Medicare (and other insurance) by hospitals, physicians and nursing homes as seen here and throughout the country.

The experiment, the methodology and the caring about patients of this small wing is yet unfolding, but as it appears now, it will be a brilliant experiment in the most American of ideals. The ideals of freedom, personal rights and dignity.

This also may eventually be corrupted elsewhere by others with less noble purpose, but it is at least a start, beyond the horrendous carnage of current practices in the existing health care system.

However, caring cannot be bought, but at least freedom and dignity can be built into a system of any kind; so can accountability and effectiveness. Perhaps this is a small model of how a larger, perhaps, a national model can be built.

It should be noted that my methodology is based on participant observation, particularly by myself and my daughter, and conversations with patients and staff.

I could add many statements made by patients which would show how my conclusions were reached, such as:

Patient:	"I don't want to go eat in the dining room?"
Nurse:	"Are you sure?"
Patient:	"Yes, I don't want to."

Nurse:	"Okay. Maybe you could try it next week."
Nurse:	"You going to eat?"
Patient:	"Yes."

Nurse:	"Do you want your dessert?"
Patient:	"No."
Nurse:	"Oh, come on, eat it."
Patient:	"No."
Nurse:	"Okay. Are you full? Is that it?"
Patient:	"Yes, I'm full."

| Speech therapist: | "$\underline{X}$ and $\underline{Y}$ don't want to participate in the group today, but they may want to next time." |

In many cases, I had to rely on physical responses of patients, since some couldn't talk clearly. As a result of this, I relied on such events as patients pushing away food, or patients disattending to events around them, or attending with apparent interest in what was going on around them.

VI. GENERAL PROBLEMS WITH THE EXISTING HEALTH CARE SYSTEM

All this is in striking contrast to the following scams (indeed crimes) encountered in our journey (my daughter and son-in-law also followed the process in horror).

An early scam, we call The Doctor Scam. We all know it. The primary physician appoints without our approval 5-6 of his peers to be specialists, who sometimes are needed, sometimes not. We assume they reciprocate the favor at other times, at very large fees. Stepping into a patient's room by any of them costs $75-$l00. This is done over and over again, at all our expense.

To add insult to injury sometimes they (the doctors) don't come, or do poor work. They still get paid.

The Hospital Scams are numerous, including: doing expensive tests over and over again, physicians giving their colleagues extra work and in general, unsavory practices. We are paying again.

Another hospital scam is forced by insurance guidlines for how long a patient can stay there. When the time comes for the patients to go, they go as soon as possible, anywhere; to the best and the worst of nursing homes or to their own homes.

Medicaid and "difficult" patients go to the worst homes.

In spite of this, the hospital scams are perhaps less heartrending than the nursing homes that receive their patients.

Yes, the hospitals in general were the best places with the best care in spite of it all, except the experimental home we will discuss.

Most of the nursing homes they go to, with the blessing of the medical and Medicare social workers and offices and administrators, are businesses. They exist to make money. To make money they cut corners on care, costs, food and facilities. To make this business work, there has to be an appearance of propriety, and the owners-managers rule with an iron hand. This is of course true of almost all institutions.

Relatives are looked at as potential troublemakers or problems and are <u>managed.</u> Those who cannot be managed easily, are managed harder. The experience of the nurse stated earlier (page 8) is an example.

This nursing home had the county and state social work organizations defending it.

They in effect defend each other and cover each other, as earlier examples documented in part. Even at the highest levels of state government, it is difficult to get action taken against even the most flagrant complaints of terrorism in a particular home.

In this case, as we have profiled, only big or powerful organizations that defend patients' rights can successfully confront <u>The System</u>.

These patients' rights organizations are usually organizations comprised of and representing patients with a particular disease. In this case it was the Huntington's Disease Association that made the difference. They were powerful enough, politically and otherwise, to be instrumental to establish the (good) model nursing home and get my wife into it.

Organizations like this are proliferating and providing a force to protect patients and it appears, to penetrate scams at all levels discussed.

<u>Organized minorities</u> appear at every level of the social world, including neighborhood organizations and racial and ethnic groups organized to protect themselves.

<u>Organized minorities</u> proliferate at the government level where special interest groups, through donations or other kinds of pressure, attempt to influence public policy in favor of their group.

Less discussed, however, may be the increasing organizations of minorities with health problems. There are hundreds of specific disease organizations that have sprung up in the last 20 or more years, from the American Cancer Society to the Huntington's Disease society discussed here, which was a powerful force in getting funds and legislation to create the demonstration unit that we are now discussing

After all, the Constitution and resulting forms of government recognize that balance of power is essential; for power alone, unchecked, is always abused. Only they thought (the founding fathers) that the structure of all society might balance power against power.

We could learn from this in creating a new structure for reformulation of national health policy.

For it is not just a matter of money, administration or power, but how it is structured and used as a system.

As we have said, the state of New Jersey provided some of the money for the "good" experiment we encountered.

The state itself appears to have become concerned, along with national government with the wasting and stealing of health money, and willing to try some experiments.

Systems of all kinds contain the seeds of their own destruction. Apparently, the old corrupt system also carried the seeds, the seeds that produced public outcry and an emptying of state and national coffers.

The general pattern is of a charismatic breakthrough by a single individual or a number of people, as in the birth of most governments and religions. After the breakthrough, the next generation organizes the new ideas into organizational and later traditional forms that are quite different from the original breakthrough period. At this point, the breakthrough ideas are altered to fit into the existing social system and are thus distorted or changed. At the same time or later the "personal interests" of the new organization begin to corrupt and perhaps work against the original breakthrough ideas.

The development of religions is a good example of this, but most charismatics in any institutional area are partially paved over by practical or personal interests.

In the face of any reforms or reorganization, there is always the recurrent problems of organization found everywhere.

Some of these problems are as follows:

1.   Careers are always involved. People in organizations protect or enhance their careers to the detriment of the organization itself, to say nothing of the formal goals of the organization.

2.   Informal organization exists everywhere, including informal goals, leaders, procedures and fun and games.

3.   The downward drift of work also is endemic especially in the health industry. Nurses' aides do the work of nurses and nurses do the work of doctors.

4.   Laziness, corruption, dishonesty and incompetence exists everywhere.

5.   The clients (or patients in this context) tend to become less important than the careers and objectives of especially the middle and upper management of any organization. In total institutions, the patients suffer as a result.

6.   The control of the organization tends to get out of the control of the owners, managers and CEO's, for a variety of reasons. One of the reasons is the sweetening of information as it rises up the organization. The CEO tends to get the "good news."

7.   Also, as we have mentioned, power tends to get in the hands of the few at the top (autocracy), and they convert organizational power to themselves and run the organization to their own desires, regardless of anyone else. And more recently, the power comes to reside in the hands of managers, not the owners, of organizations. These managers serve not the owners or their purposes, but rather, the manager's enrichment. Thus we see a national picture of the new Managerial Capitalism and Managerial Politics in government. This seems increasingly the case in post-industrial societies where a number of different managerial and professional elites compete against each other.

So, with the best of intentions and new structures all organizations including "the experiment" just discussed may be subject to the forces listed above, and must be continually overseen by all of us. In this case (medical organization), the large patient rights-single disease organizations seem to be our best protection, but they too can be corrupted by the same desire for money, power and position they set out to fight.

Nevertheless, there is a public outcry and a mass movement to merge the "experiment" with new systems of health care at all levels. It will probably succeed since at least one-fourth of the population by the year 2000 will be over 50, and they and their children are greatly concerned. This "experiment" is just a tip of the iceberg.

It is significant to notice that America is the only advanced democracy in the world that does not have some kind of socialized medicine, where some kind of decent care is available to all. Even Cuba provides this.

What is wrong here?
What is the reason?

VII. CONTRASTING NURSING HOMES

For those of you who are of an analytical mind, we can contrast the first two nursing homes with the final one.

The first nursing home was (unintentionally?) destructive, but not degradational, with some love, exchange, and intimacy.[1]

The second and <u>worst</u>, if we wish to take a <u>moral</u> position or a practical position (often a contradiction in logic), consisted mostly of destructive (often intentional) degradational (often intentional), no love, no intimacy, no exchange or anything else that could be positive, etc.[2]

The third and final nursing home - the experiment - is largely engaged in love, intimacy, therapeutic and not intentionally or even <u>very</u> destructive or degradational.

This is not to say we did not meet nurses and aides in the first two nursing homes that provided love, therapy, intimacy and exchange. We did find these people going out of their way in spite of the circumstances.

Again, we found physicians who were not destructive, degradational, and at worst did not have the technical logic (expertise) to do good work or worked in organizational settings where the emphasis tended to be placed on exchange and political logics[3] (making money and avoiding suits).

Nurses, in general, were also some of the best of the lot, who were usually technically competent, and often caring.

---

[1]See James H. Parker, *Social Logics: Conversations and Groups in Everyday Life*, University Press of America (Lanham. MD and London, England), 1985, esp. pp. 1-28 and 51-66, and *Logics II: The Sociobiology of Social and Other Logics*, University Press of America, 1992, also written by James H. Parker.

[2]Op. cit.

[3]Op. cit.

The aides were apparently caught in a low-paying occupation, doing the "dirty work," who usually but not always were alienated from their work. As a result of this, the aides used less technical (expertise), and were often involved in escape logic,[4] avoiding work, patients, and just looked at TV or slept in patients' rooms.

Having trained future social workers myself (not M.S.W. degrees, but B.A. degrees), I somewhat understand the lower level social workers (B.A.'s). They're often not well enough trained or with sufficient commitment to their jobs, so as a result, turn into bureaucrats adapting a strictly bureaucratic logic[5] (strategies?) which was often less than helpful.

The second level social workers (Masters of Social Work degrees) have a good deal more specialized training, are better paid, etc., so show a different profile. They (the M.S.W.'s) usually are technically competent, tend to care for (love logic, therapeutic and intimacy logic[6]) their patients and clients. They are also a bright spot in an otherwise dismal picture.

The conclusion (or correlation) seems to be that the better the training (M.D.'s, M.S.W.'s, R.N.'s, etc.) the better the care they provide - it is obviously not always true - but there is a high correlation between education and competence and maybe even caring about patients.

The unsung heroes or heroines are many. They do their job in spite of the worst circumstances, they can be found throughout the health system, and even in everyday life. They make care positive and meaningful.

No system, social or technical can suppress these loving, unsung heroes. For they persist, endowing the worst place with love, intimacy and meaning, along with a bit of the comedic and polite sociability.[7]

This also tends to be true of everyday life, in general, among ordinary people.

---

[4]Op. cit.

[5]Op. cit.

[6]Op. cit.

[7]Op. cit.

VIII. THE PICNIC AND THE HALLOWEEN PARTY

It was organized as freedom eventually becomes. The patients, their loved ones, the nurses, the aides, the social workers and some of their children were there on a September picnic in a park across from the "home." Some laid on blankets in the sun. There was food on a long table which everybody brought. There was enough for everyone. There were activities like the volleyball game where almost everybody participated; young, old, sick, the helpers, the black, the white, the poor, the better off and so forth.

The volleyball game began, and most everyone was a part of it, even the four-year-old's. A certain excitement and oneness and spontaneous joy unfolded beyond any good scientific description, beyond words. It was the utopia which all seek, even for a few moments, of sharing joy and caring, and it was beyond anything except just being there.

It was fun that time, a utopia for everybody where there was no old or young, or sick or well, or any other distinction. Everybody was equal, and nobody owned each other but just were being with each other in joy (which can only happen sometimes). For an hour or two, we knew what utopia could be.

It was an example of the unfolding of freedom and caring and love at this place where there are rules and procedures. But the experiment in freedom for everybody was working.

It was, however, beyond words, other than to say it was in Maslow's terms a peak experience of a group of people, who probably will not forget it.

They decided (everybody) they would do it again on Christmas - but it would be on the "inside", somebody jokingly announced.

I look with anticipation toward Christmas - when hopefully there will be joy again and something we all could share.

* * *

Later that fall there was a Halloween party at the nursing home.

* * *

It is difficult to turn tragedy into comedy. A few writers have done it, such as Dante in *The Inferno* in *The Divine Comedy.*

The nursing home and its Huntington's patients, without any doubt, looked at Halloween as their favorite holiday. Why this is so, I do not know, except that it seems to transform the theme of death and suffering into comedy and laughter (much like the picnic in some ways).

The day before the Halloween celebration, my daughter and myself visited my wife. We were greeted with signs saying "Blood Bank" and "Brain Donations", obviously a comic attempt to transform death into a holiday. We might say that one title of this holiday could be *Death Takes a Holiday.* There were skeletons hanging by their necks and spiderwebs with large spiders in the corners. The notice earlier sent to us about the event to come had a picture of "bobbing for apples" by the patients, who of course would find that difficult, if not impossible, to do.

In any case, the patients were excited by the prospect of the comedy and celebration of ghouls, ghosts, the living dead and so on.

My wife was asked by my daughter about Halloween. She (my wife) was excited by just the word. Asked if she wanted a costume, as she lay there peacefully, she said, "Yes...yes, I want one."

"A costume?"

"Yes."

"What kind, Mom?"

"Anything."

"How about a witch costume with a black hat?"

"Yes...yes," she said, getting more enthusiastic.

So we went out and got a witch costume and brought it back. She was delighted.

"Do you like it?"

"Yes...I do."

"You want to be a witch?"

"Yes. I like the costume."

She was more excited than she had been for months, as were the other patients who knew what was going on.

As (my daughter and I) left the place, I said, "The whole place looks like Halloween already."

Yes, it always does, with the crippled bodies and people walking like those in *The Night of the Living Dead.*

"Some of them are already practically dead."

"Yes, I know."

But in any case, at Halloween and during the week before it, tragedy becomes comedy, almost like Dante's *Inferno*, at least Ciardi's translation. Only here, the playing out of the actual daily Halloween, sickness, suffering, deformity and death become a cause for celebration.

I couldn't go to the actual party, but if possible I shall get a firsthand report of the event, with all its color, humor and laughing in the face of death. The comedic, at least, can overcome the tragic, here and elsewhere.

Although, as I have said, I was not able to be at the Halloween party itself, from all reports it was a great success. Both patients and staff enjoyed the celebration. Patients were dressed in costumes, as were some of the staff. There *was* bobbing for apples, a nice dinner (with throwing or dropping of food) and a general air of festivity. Everyone was potentially (in the long run, at least) going to be sick and dead, and were facing it with humor and lack of grace. It didn't matter if they were Christian, or Jewish or anything else. As in the picnic, it didn't matter how old they were, what sex they were or their race or ethnic background.

It was like the picnic, except this was a celebration of the inevitable, assisted by the traditions of ghouls, ghosts and disguised identities with masks and costumes.

Much fun was had by all, even perhaps by those who were practically brain dead and unaware, for it was a *celebration* of what they already were: virtually dead.

The party and the holiday in general, all over, provided a *framework* in which to view the inevitable for everyone, namely death. But it was and is a framework that did not speak of redemption, faith or the normal religious themes.

Instead it was a fantasy framework which included centuries of secular celebration of these matters. Ghosts could be seen as real or not (e.g., Shakespeare, *Hamlet*). Spirits could be seen as real or not (e.g., Shakespeare, *A Midsummer Night's Dream*). Death itself could be seen as real or not (e.g., funerals in all cultures, and also by religions in all cultures). And as with Shakespeare and Dante and the rest of the great writers, suffering and death could be seen as *serious or not.*

So the framwork of Halloween, here as elsewhere, includes among other things a *denial of death*, or at least laughing in the face of it, or rationalizing through mythic ritual the reality or the non-reality of it.

For this place (the nursing home), every day was Halloween in a sense. Some patients denied death, some (all?) patients wore masks the year round (e.g., *The Masque of the Red Death*, and the general view that we all wear masks).

Oddly enough, even the sickest patients, throughout the year, tried and usually succeeded in wearing some kind of social mask, even the mask of death at the end, adjusted by the mortician: peaceful, beautiful and even socially proper.

The mask of many Huntington's patients, although distorted by their disease many times, is constantly being re-set in proper place and proper demeanor, sometimes with the help of the staff. This is so even at the end or near the end, in sickness and in health, in the sickest of people, as personally and socially required.

Some deviants, however, here and in ordinary society, drop their masks and show what's underneath, to the horror and disgust of everybody, and thereby constitute a great threat to our fictional identities which we have come to believe in, at least in part, and have become part of our world view and personal view of ourselves and our defenses and strategies.

Here (in the nursing home) as elsewhere, when one is very sick, a very great fear on the part of the patient is that they cannot *control* their masks, their sustained conventional interactions with others, to the extent that they do not want to see people or be seen (much) by them. This of course is that case with us all, except the social deviant who doesn't care anymore and has gone beyond shame and guilt and social convention.

Thus the Halloween party was instructive, to me, at the very least, about part of the human condition, of masks, of fantasies, of laughter, of death and social convention and social identity of the well and the sick.

* * *

The day before the party, when I was there at the home, I had an article from *The New York Times* Science section, and it was rapidly reproduced and passed around among the staff and probably the patients, for the article was essentially about a very probable scientific treatment and cure for this particular disease.

I understand that at the Halloween party a few people, staff and patients, attempted to dance with the music. I was told that one patient approached a staff member and said, "Could I have the last dance?" and the staff member reportedly replied, "Yes, but I'm sure this is not your last dance, and did you see the article?"

The patient said, "No," and danced anyway.

IX. IS FREEDOM WORKING?

(I think freedom is working.)

It was existential. It was experimental. It was not a system that happened. In 1960's terms, it was a <u>Happening</u> - that can only be experienced and cannot really be talked about as a <u>systemic occurrence</u>, but only vaguely as a very loose systemic success.

The existential problem of being - sick or well - had been breached, and all patients and staff were together trying to find joy amidst the suffering.

The organization of events during a given month is fairly typical. Paraphrasing one monthly schedule, we find:

1. Church services and events (which seem very frequent).
2. Bingo and other group games.
3. Trips to baseball games, to the pool and other outside places.
4. Group therapy of various kinds (speech, socio-emotional, musical, recreational, physical).

There is, however, more or less free time when the patients can watch TV, walk around the halls and talk to each other.

In the case of this nursing home, the events really happened for the benefit of the patients. It looks a lot like other places, doesn't it? But it isn't.

I also received the following in the mail which I will subsequently report on, as another side of the experiment in freedom and the medical model, I guess you could say.

```
                              9/4/91
Dear Dr. Parker:

      Interdisciplinary Committee Meetings, during which
staff members from each department and discipline meet
to discuss each Huntington's Disease patient's progress
and therapeutic goals, are scheduled for Alice Parker on
Wednesday, 9/11/91, at 2:15 p.m.   We welcome your
participation and hope that you will be able to attend.
Please call either ... to let us know if you plan to
attend.

      We look forward to hearing from you.

                        Very truly yours,


                        Social Worker - HD Unit
```

There was a certain tenseness as the social workers and nurses sat around the table - who worked with her (the patient) every day.

There was also a certain sadness amongst them as they recounted the decline of the patient and how they couldn't do much about it. It was like resignation to hear of death at least of the body and seeing the patient dying in spite of their efforts.

So they would just try to make her as comfortable as possible, not understanding her recent behavior.

"If I understand right, what we are seeing is the natural progress of the disease," I said.

"Yes ... yes," they said as one.

"Do you have any suggestions?" a social worker asked.

"Well," I replied, "she probably can use some Valium or something like that to calm her down."

"Yes, but," one social worker said, "part of the philosophy here is to not sedate anymore than necessary."

"I understand," I said.

"Yes, the policy is freedom and natural life as much as possible." They continued, "Even though patients scream and hit each other, and act really crazy sometimes."

It seemed though that medically the limits of freedom and natural living were being pressed hard.

For they need to protect to some extent patients from each other's hostility and rages. So they did their best with a minimum of restraint, and they needed to give some medicine just so the patients could even move and eat correctly, which was difficult. On the faces of these health professionals you could still see caring, but tiredness and some sad resignation about the inevitability of the "patient's progress."

They still cared but they could do little but hold back the inevitable a little bit.

We discussed freedom and dignity for a while and decided that some physical restraints were at times necessary, and that they would look into the possibility of Valium to calm her down.

Yet in spite of all this, the ideals had not died. The practicality of patient management had come to the fore - to compromise the ideals of freedom and natural living.

But there comes a time and it comes to everybody that others must take care of you and the balance between freedom and practicality (even for the good of the patient) takes place and death and disease progress. Hopefully, in this experiment, they will die with dignity and a sense of self worth and in the midst of caring individuals.

There lies the dilemma of a health system, any health system - whether it be in the person's own home or in an impersonal hospital. The issue of freedom and control meets us at the very end, and at every turn.

Again, we are reminded of the "Official" rights of the residents which this nursing home meets and exceeds.

* * *

BILL OF RIGHTS*

Each resident shall be entitled to the following rights:

*   State of New Jersey, Department of Health

1. To retain the services of a physician the patient chooses, at the patient's own expense or through a health care plan.

2. To have a physician explain to the patient, in language that the patient understands, his or her complete medical condition, the recommended treatment, and the expected results of the treatment. If this information would be detrimental to the patient's health, the explanation must be provided to his or her next of kin or guardian and documented in the patient's medical record.

3. To participate, to the fullest extent that the patient is able, in planning his or her own medical treatment and care.

4. To refuse medication and treatment after the patient has been informed, in language that the patient understands, of the possible consequences of this decision. The patient may also refuse to participate in experimental research, including the investigations of new drugs and medical devices. The patient will be included in experimental research only when he or she gives informed, written consent to such participation.

5. To be free from physical and mental abuse. The resident may file a complaint with the state survey and certification agency concerning resident abuse, neglect, and misappropriation of resident property.

6. To be free from chemical and physical restraints, unless they are authorized by a physician for a limited period of time to protect the patient or others from injury. Under no circumstances will the patient be confined in a locked room or restrained for punishment, for the convenience of the nursing home staff, or with the use of excessive drug dosages.

7. To manage his or her own finances or to have that responsibility delegated to a family member, an assigned guardian, the nursing home administrator, or some other individual with power of attorney. The patient's

authorization must be in writing, and must be witnessed in writing.

8.   To receive a written statement describing the services provided by the nursing home and the related charges. This statement must also include the nursing home's policies for payment of fees, deposits, and refunds. The patient must receive this statement prior to or at the time of admission, and afterward whenever there are any changes.

9.   To receive a quarterly written account of all patient's funds and itemized property that are deposited with the facility for the patient's use and safekeeping. This record must also show the amount of property in the account at the beginning and end of the accounting period, as well as a list of all deposits and withdrawals, substantiated by receipts given to the patient or his or her guardian. Patient's fund will be kept in an interest bearing account. The individual financial record is available on request to the resident or his or her legal representative.

10. To have daily access during specified hours to the money and property that the patient has deposited with the nursing home. The patient also may delegate this right of access to his or her representative.

11. To live in safe, decent, and clean conditions in a nursing home that does not admit more residents than it can safely accommodate while providing adequate nursing care.

12. To be treated with courtesy, consideration, and respect for the patient's dignity and individuality. The nursing home may not move the patient to a different bed or room in the facility if the relocation is arbitrary and capricious.

13. To wear his or her own clothes, unless this would be unsafe or impractical. All clothes provided by the nursing home must fit in a way that is not demeaning to the patient.

14. To keep and use his or her personal property, unless this would be unsafe, impractical, or an infringement on the

rights of other residents. The nursing home must take precautions to ensure that the patient's personal possessions are secure from theft, loss and misplacement.

15. To have physical privacy. The patient must be allowed, for example, to maintain the privacy of his or her body during medical treatment and personal hygiene activities, such as bathing and using the toilet, unless the patient needs assistance for his or her own safety.

16. To have reasonable opportunities for private and intimate physical and social interaction with other people, including arrangements for privacy when the patient's spouse visits. If the patient and his or her spouse are both residents of the same nursing home, they must be given the opportunity to share a room, unless this is medically inadvisable, as documented in their records by a physician.

17. To have confidential treatment of information about the patient. Information in the patient's records shall not be released to anyone outside the nursing home without the patient's approval, unless the patient transfers to another health care facility, or unless the release of the information is required by law, a third-party payment contract, or the New Jersey State Department of Health. The resident has the right to inspect and purchase photocopies of all records pertaining to the resident upon written request and 48 hours notice to the facility.

18. To receive and send mail in unopened envelopes, unless the patient requests otherwise. The patient also has a right to request and receive assistance in reading and writing correspondence unless it is medically contraindicated.

19. To have access to a telephone without anyone deliberately listening to the conversation, and, if technically feasible, to have a private telephone in his or her living quarters at the patient's own expense.

20. To stay out of bed as long as the patient desires and to be awakened for routine daily care no more than two hours

before breakfast is served, unless a physician recommends otherwise and specifies the reasons in the patient's medical record.

21. To receive assistance in awakening, getting dressed, and participating in the facility's activities, unless a physician specifies reasons in the patient's medical record.

22. To meet with any visitors of the resident's choice between 8:00 a.m. and 8:00 p.m. daily. If the resident is critically ill, he or she may receive visits at any time from next of kin or a guardian, unless a physician documents that this would be harmful to the resident's health.

23. To take part in nursing home activities, and to meet with and participate in the activities of any social, religious, and community groups, as long as these activities do not disrupt the lives of other residents.

24. To leave the nursing home during the day with the approval of a physician and with the resident's whereabouts noted on a sign-out record. Arrangements may also be made with the nursing home for an absence overnight or longer.

25. To refuse to perform services for the nursing home.

26. To request visits at any time by representatives of the religion of the resident's choice and, upon the resident's request, to attend outside religious services at his or her own expense. No religious beliefs or practices may be imposed on any resident.

27. To participate in meals, recreation, and social activities without being subjected to discrimination based on age, race, religion, sex and nationality, or disability. The patient's participation may be restricted or prohibited only upon the written recommendation of his or her physician.

28. To organize and participate in a Resident Council that presents residents' concerns to the administrator of the facility.

29.   To discharge himself or herself from the nursing home by presenting a release signed by the resident. If the resident is an adjudicated mental incompetent, the release must be signed by his or her next of kin or guardian.

30.   To be transferred or discharged only for one or more of the following reasons and the reason for the transfer or discharge must be recorded in the patient's medical record.
        I.   In an emergency, with notification of the patient's physician and next of kin or guardian.
        II.   For medical reasons or to protect the patient's welfare or the welfare of others.
        III.   For nonpayment of fees, in situations not prohibited by law.
        IV.   Because the resident's health has improved sufficiently so the resident no longer needs the facility's services.

31.   To receive written notice at least 30 days in advance when the nursing home requests the patient's transfer or discharge, except in an emergency. Written notice must also be provided to the patient's next of kin or guardian 30 days in advance.

32.   To be given a written statement of all patient rights as well as any additional regulations established by the nursing home involving patient rights and responsibilities. The nursing home shall require each patient or his or her guardian to sign a copy of this document. In addition, a copy must be posted in a conspicuous, public place in the nursing home. Copies must also be given to the patient's next of kin and distributed to staff members. The nursing home is responsible for developing and implementing policies to protect patient rights.

33.   To retain and exercise all the constitutional, civil, and legal rights to which the patient is entitled by law. The nursing home must encourage and help each patient to exercise these rights.

34.   To voice complaints without being threatened or punished.

(a)   Each patient is entitled to complain and present his or her grievances to the nursing home administrator and staff, to government agencies, and to anyone else without fear of interference, discharge, or reprisal. The nursing home is required to provide each patient and his and or next of kin or guardian with the names, addresses, and telephone numbers of the government agencies to which a patient can complain and ask questions, including the New Jersey State Department of Health and the Office of the Ombudsman for the Institutionalized Elderly. These names, addresses, and telephone numbers must be posted in a conspicuous place near every public telephone and on all public bulletin boards in the nursing home.

(b)   Each patient, patient's next of kin, and patient's guardian shall be informed of the patient rights enumerated in this subchapter, and each shall be explained to him or her. None of these rights shall be abridged or violated by the facility or any of its staff.

35.   A resident has the right to examine the results of the most recent survey of the facility conducted by Federal or State surveyors and any plan of correction in effect with respect to the facility. The results will be posted in the facility.

36.   A resident has the right to receive information from agencies acting as client advocates, and be afforded the opportunity to contact these agencies.

37.   A resident has the right to self administer drugs unless the interdisciplinary team has determined for each resident that this practice is unsafe.

38.   A resident has the right to receive notice before the resident's room or roommate in the facility change.

39.   The resident has the right and the facility must provide immediate access to any resident by the following:
    I.   Any representative of the secretary
    II.   Any representative of the state
    III.   The resident's individual system

IV. The state long-term care ombudsman
V. The agency responsible for the protection and advocacy system for developmentally disabled individuals.
VI. The agency responsible for the protection and advocacy system for mentally ill individuals.

40. Except in a medical emergency or when a resident is incompetent, a facility must consult with the resident immediately and notify the resident's physician; and if unknown, the resident's legal representative or interested family member within 24 hours when there is:

I. An accident involving the resident which results in injury;
II. A significant change in the resident's physical, mental, or psychosocial status;
III. A need to alter treatment significantly; or
IV. A decision to transfer or discharge the resident from the facility as specified in 483.12(a).

X. THE FREEDOM TO DIE

The ultimate freedom is now being offered to residents of the home. That is, the freedom to decide when they will die.

The nursing home offers relatives and friends a session in which the problems and possibilities of a "living will" will be discussed, which will then be discussed with the patient. A living will is a statement by the patient how, whether and when he or she wishes to die. This is in the ultimate sense, the ultimate freedom. This is not a suicide pact, but a well spelled-out statement of when and if artificial life support systems may be turned off or initiated.

I have already discussed this with my wife and she said, "It's up to you." She has been declared incompetent to sign a living will. What a responsibility, what a problem, for when the time comes she will not be able to speak or write or may not be in her right mind. I, myself, would prefer if she took this final act of freedom and responsibility onto herself. Perhaps her social workers will talk to her about this. I feel depressed, myself, by this fact, for I have a responsibility over the life or death of my own wife. Maybe something can be worked out. Who knows?

This is not freedom for me, it is responsibility for myself and others. But how far does responsibility go, to what extent, and is there a point in modern medicine where it becomes a social responsibility in terms of the cost of keeping people alive?

She has seemed at times to want to live as long as possible, but has also stated, "I want to die, I want to die." I guess I should respect her wishes, but her wishes seem to alternate. But it seems also her wish that "I" be ultimately trusted and responsible at some critical point, perhaps when she is for all purposes dead except for the beating of the heart and faint brain waves. I don't know, if this freedom is beginning to impinge on me, as more, almost unbearable responsibility. How in a larger sense she has not used her freedom to ask for "life as long as possible," although she has sometimes seemed uncertain.

They are talking about feeding her directly into the stomach, under which conditions she would "live?" a normal life span, for people do not die from this disease, but usually die of pneumonia caused by bits of food coughed into the lungs or choking.

Herein lies the problem: I will respect her wishes, but I'm not sure what they are.

As far as what is natural or unnatural living, which is a high priority of the nursing home, is a difficult point. It seems to be their emerging position to at least give the option of letting the patient decide what is natural or unnatural. This of course is a kind of ultimate freedom also, but one for which the families, the society, must pay.

A decision like this about freedom does have consequences and all sorts of ramifications, especially for the question of quality of life vs. quantity of life, and it raises questions of who should get how much of medical care, for it is limited in quantity and quality and it costs society many resources. These questions about individual freedom are difficult, for as always, the individual's freedom rushes headlong into the needs and freedom of others; in this case the needs for health care for others.

Anyway, we, the society, are in the process of working out an equitable balance between the inexorable and continuing problem of the individual vs. the society - or the needs of the individual vs. the needs of the society. Freedom is always at issue and also justice and love.

* * * * *

I went to the meeting where they discussed the Living Will and lack of it.

It was some consolation, but not much.

We saw a clinically pure video about medical ethics which lasted about half an hour dealing with life and death decisions.

The social worker who was nice enough, asked if there were any questions and there were a few. Everybody looked a little tired and befuddled by the complexities of deciding how and when to die, either for others or for themselves.

We all had cake and coffee and a few talked and quickly drifted off to their respective homes.

I ate another piece of cake and visited my wife who was lying down ready to go to sleep. She seemed calm and happy to see me and I felt she was aware enough but I could <u>not</u> ask her again under what conditions she wanted to die.

I could not do it, at that time anyway. So I just talked for a while and she said she was glad to see me and finally I had the courage to say, "Do you want them to artificially feed you through a tube into your stomach?" She said "No." She just looked at me and I said goodbye, kissed her and left for home, still not knowing exactly what she wanted, but I was pretty sure.

On the way home I felt good somehow, for at least I had some idea of the way things were to evolve.

In one last effort to avoid the responsibility for somebody else's freedom, I asked my daughter when I got there.

"Is it okay if I decide this question?"

"What question?"

"Whether she should be on an artificial life support system for perhaps 20 years?"

"No, she shouldn't," she said. And we both watched TV, for an hour.

I don't remember the program but we were both quiet not needing to talk for it would have been, at that time, an intrusion on each of us and our sense of having said something real to each other, however painful or final.

There probably never had been something so final for either of us. As with most important decisions, you make them yourself, or somebody does it for you.

It simply wasn't, and never is, clear what the "somebody else" would do.

Nevertheless, the experiment was proceeding patiently and lovingly toward the issue of death.

Walking us through the steps before it happened was the most freedom they could give, and they gave it in a quiet peace of accepting finality and destiny.

However, as I said previously, I had become a decider of destiny. We were urged at that quiet meeting to consider that any of us, no matter how young or old, could be in that precarious position of not being able, in a coma or some other state, to decide how and when we would die.

So quietly, so calm was the short speech by the director of social work, that death was just an extension of life not to be feared for it would come to us all, but to be a quiet final decision, who should decide, ourselves in a Living Will, or a loved one, or somebody else who knew us not, except as people in serious trouble medically and was it worth saving us.

I felt like I had gone to a funeral like Albert Camus, quietly and without passion, just gone to a funeral that might not happen for 20 years.

It was very existential and even philosophical but the freedom was being assigned to me in place of somebody else's freedom.

Again, the experiment did not evade the "realities" of the situation of the patients and their families. They did just what they started out to do; give away freedom to those who needed or wanted it. In this case, we were not sure we wanted this much freedom, for as always freedom entails responsibilities on somebody's part.

The somebody now was us.

We had another meeting of the unplanned support group, for which they had nothing planned.

But at last, ever since the Picnic, that September, that being together from all walks of life was enough then, and it might be again.

At least we would have the freedom not to have to do or say anything in particular - sort of a purposeless freedom never ending, from generation to generation, as it were.

They said at that fatal meeting, that if the patient was not competent to sign a Living Will, the guardian, me, would have to carry out his or her wishes. (Later they said, with the help of an ethics committee.)

How interesting - death by committee.

I knew when they said this that it would not just be one decision, but many decisions over the course of years. So, my freedom would be exercised again and again, and even afterwards doubt would remain.

Also, we as guardians or anyone else live in a social world that makes judgments, long after you've gone, as to how well or whether you should have made such a life and death decision. I know because I've seen it happen. You have freedom, unfortunately, in a social context, as if it were not enough that you had to make a decision at all and live with it.

This experiment in freedom has landed on my shoulders. They (the nursing home) has said in effect, "Now you make decisions about freedom and dignity, and life and death for another, and furthermore, make a big decision, with a Living Will, how and when you want to die."

What a responsibility. And it goes on and on, for given this new freedom, some person, unless I'm hit by a truck, will have to make a series of decisions about my life and death.

As the technology, especially the new genetic medicine proceeds further, people will live, perhaps say some, to 140 years old.

What kinds of decisions will the society have to make when this happens? I suspect, although I do not know, that the Freedom to Live will become very problematic as the average age increases and people can be kept alive longer and longer; another problem for freedom and the necessity to make decisions as to "under what conditions should people be allowed to live?"

I guess we will just have to wait and see.

But as usual there will be some limits to Freedom of the Individual to Live when it collides with the needs of the collective will.

Ethics indeed will enter medicine with full force, as it is beginning to do now, with the coming of age of medical ethicists -and life and death debated in philosophy departments, as well as in the medical field.

But the problems we have with this issue now are quite enough, and now that most states allow Living Wills, for the time being people are being urged to make a decision early about The Quality of Life they want to end life with.

It is now a question of Quality vs. Quantity among medical ethicists and others, including the rest of us. Many of the very young are now saying, "I don't want to live to be 80 or 90 or 100. I don't want to be fed by a tube."

What will they say when they are 80 or 90? Many people are opting apparently for a more or less healthy and painless end to life.

But this remains to be seen.

XI. THE LIVING WILL

Included below is sort of a final Declaration of Independence for a patient, but still involves trust, love and caring.

Planning Ahead For Your Health Care:
Making Your Wishes Known*

The purpose of this brochure is to help you prepare an advance directive which reflects your wishes concerning medical care. While it contains sample forms and directions, advance directives are very personal documents and you should feel free to develop one which best suits your own needs. The brochure consists of the following parts:
1. Introduction
2. Questions and Answers
3. Terms You Should Understand
4. Sample Forms
5. Checklist
6. Wallet size I.D. cards (inside back cover)

1. Introduction:
Why this booklet?

As Americans, we take it for granted that we are entitled to make decisions about our own health care. Most of the time we make these decisions after talking with our own physician about the advantages and disadvantages of various treatment options. The right of a competent individual to accept or refuse medical treatment is a fundamental right protected by law.

*A publication of the New Jersey Bioethics Commission, 1991

But what happens if serious illness, injury or permanent loss of mental capacity makes us incapable of talking to a doctor and deciding what medical treatments we do or do not want? These situations pose difficult questions to all of us as patients, family members, friends and health care professionals. Who makes these decisions if we can't make them for ourselves? If we can't make our preferences known how can we be sure that our wishes will be respected? If disagreements arise among those caring for us about different treatment alternatives how will they be resolved? Is there a way to alleviate the burdens shouldered by family members and loved ones when critical medical decisions must be made?

By using documents known as **advance directives for health care,** you can answer some of these questions and give yourself the security of knowing that you can continue to have a say in your own treatment. A properly prepared **advance directive** permits you to plan ahead so you can both make your wishes known, and select someone who will see to it that your wishes are followed.

After all, if you are seriously ill or injured and can't make decisions for yourself someone will have to decide about your medical care. Doesn't it make sense to

- Have a person you trust make decisions for you, or

- Provide instructions about the treatment you do and do not want, or

- Both. Appoint a person to make decisions **and** provide them with instructions.

A Few Definitions

Throughout this booklet we're going to use four phrases. Each of these phrases has a special meaning when it comes to allowing you to make decisions about your future health care.

- **Advance directive**--If you want your wishes to guide those responsible for your care you have to plan for what you want in advance. Generally such planning is more likely to be effective if it's done in writing. So, by an "advance directive" we mean any written instructions you prepare in advance to say what kind of medical care you want in the event you become unable to make decisions for yourself.

There are three kinds of advance directives:

1.   **Proxy directives**--One way to have a say in your future medical care is to designate a person (a proxy) you trust and give that person the legal authority to decide for you if you are unable to make decisions for yourself. Your chosen proxy (known as a **health care representative**) serves as your substitute, "standing in" for you in discussions with your physician and others responsible for your care. So, by a **proxy directive** we mean written directions that name a "proxy" to act for you. Another term some people use for a proxy directive is a "durable power of attorney for health care."

2.   **Instruction directives**--Another way to have a say in your future medical care is to provide those responsible for your care with a statement of your medical treatment preferences. By **"instruction directive"** we mean written directions that spell out in advance what medical treatment you wish to accept or refuse and the circumstances in which you want your wishes implemented. These instructions then serve as a guide to those responsible for your care. Another term some people use for an instruction directive is a "living will".

3.   **Combined directives**--A third way combines features of both the **proxy** and the **instruction directive.** You may prefer to give both written instructions, and to designate a health care representative or proxy to see that your instructions are carried out. So, by a **"combined directive"** we mean a single document in which you select a health care representative and provide him or her with a statement of your medical treatment preferences.

Whichever form you choose, it is important to remember to discuss your health care preferences with others. In order to help you choose the kind of directive which best suits your circumstances, the following pages answer some frequently asked questions about advance directives.

2.   Questions and Answers

Why should I consider writing an advance directive?

Serious injury, illness or mental incapacity may make it impossible for you to make health care decisions for yourself. In these situations, those responsible for your care will have to make decisions for you. Advance directives are legal documents which provide information about your treatment preferences to those caring for you, helping to insure that your wishes are respected even when you can't make decisions for yourself. A clearly written directive helps prevent disagreements among those close to you and alleviates some of the burdens of decision-making which are often experienced by family members, friends and health care providers.

When does my advance directive take effect?

Your directive takes effect when you no longer have the ability to make decisions about your health care. This judgment is normally made by your attending physician, and any additional physicians who may be required by law to examine you. If there is any doubt about your ability to make such decisions, your doctor will consult with another doctor with training and experience in this area. Together they will decide if you are unable to make your own health care decisions.

What happens if I regain the ability to make my own decisions?

If you regain your ability to make decisions, then you resume making your own decisions directly. Your directive is in effect only as long as you are unable to make your own decisions.

What is the advantage of having a health care representative, isn't it enough to have an instruction directive?

Your doctor and other health care professionals are legally obligated to consider your expressed wishes as stated in your **instruction directive** or "living will". However, instances may occur in which medical circumstances arise or treatments are proposed that you may not have thought about when you wrote your directive. If this happens your **health care representative** has the authority to participate in discussions with your health care providers and to make treatment decisions for you in accordance with what he or she knows of your wishes. Your health care representative will also be able to make decisions as your medical condition changes, in accordance with your wishes and best interests.

If I decide to appoint a health care representative, who should I trust with this task?

The person you choose to be your health care representative has the legal right to accept or refuse medical treatment (including life-sustaining measures) on your behalf and to assure that your wishes concerning your medical treatment are carried out. You should choose a person who knows you well, and who is familiar with your feelings about different types of medical treatment and the conditions under which you would choose to accept or refuse either a specific treatment or all treatment.

A health care representative must understand that his or her responsibility is to implement your wishes even if your representative or others might disagree with them. So it is important to select someone in whose judgement you have confidence. People that you might consider asking to be your health care representative include:

- a member of your family or a very close friend, your priest, rabbi, or minister, or

- a trusted health care provider, but your attending physician cannot serve as both your physician and your health care representative.

Should I discuss my wishes with my health care representative and others?

Absolutely!   Your health care representative is the person who speaks for you when you can't speak for yourself. It is very important that he or she has a clear sense of your feelings, attitudes and health care preferences. You should also discuss your wishes with your physician, family members and others who will be involved in caring for you.

Does my health care representative have the authority to make all health care decisions for me?

It is up to you to say what your health care representative can and cannot decide. You may wish to give him or her broad authority to make all treatment decisions including decisions to forego life-sustaining measures. On the other hand, you may wish to restrict the authority to specific treatments or circumstances. Your representative has to respect those limitations.

Is my doctor obligated to talk to my health care representative?

Yes.   Your health care representative has the legal authority to make medical decisions on your behalf, in consultation with your doctor. Your doctor is legally obligated to consult with your chosen representative and to respect his or her decision as if it were your decision.

Is my health care representative the only person who can speak for me, or can other friends or family members participate in making treatment decisions?

It is generally a good idea for your health care representative to consult with family members or others in making decisions, and if you wish you can direct that he or she do so. It should be understood by everyone, however, that your health care representative is the only person with the legal authority to make decisions about your health care even if others disagree.

If I want to give specific instructions about my medical care, what should I say?

If you have any special concerns about particular treatments, you should clearly express them in your directive. If you feel there are medical conditions which would lead you to decide to forego all medical treatment, including life-sustaining measures, and accept an earlier death, this should be clearly indicated in your directive.

Are there particular treatments I should specifically mention in my directive?

It is a good idea to indicate your specific preferences concerning two specific kinds of life-sustaining measures: artificially provided fluids and nutrition and cardiopulmonary resuscitation. Stating your preferences clearly concerning these two treatments will be of considerable help in avoiding uncertainty, disagreements or confusion about your wishes. The enclosed forms provide a space for you to state specific directions concerning your wishes with respect to these two forms of treatment.

Can I request all measures be taken to sustain my life?

Yes. You should make this choice clear in your advance directive. Remember, a directive can be used to request medical treatments as well as to refuse unwanted ones.

Does my doctor have to carry out my wishes as stated in my instruction directive?

If your treatment preferences are clear your doctor is legally obligated to implement your wishes, unless doing this would violate his or her conscience or accepted medical practice. If your doctor is unwilling to honor your wishes he or she must assist in transferring you to the care of another doctor.

Can I make changes in my directive?

Yes. An advance directive can be updated or modified, in whole or in part, at any time, by a legally competent individual. You should update your directive whenever you feel it no longer accurately reflects your wishes. It is a good idea to review your directive on a regular basis, perhaps every 5 years. Each time you review the directive, indicate the date on the form itself and have someone witness the changes you make. If you make a lot of changes, you may want to write a new directive. Remember to notify all those important to you of any changes you make.

Can I revoke my directive at any time?

Yes. You can revoke your directive at any time, regardless of your physical or mental condition. This can be done in writing, orally, or by any action which indicates that you no longer want the directive to be in effect.

Who should have copies of my advance directive?

A copy should be given to the person that you have named as your health care representative, as well as to your family, your doctor and others who are important to you. If you enter a hospital, nursing home, or hospice, a copy of your advance directive should be provided so that it can be made part of your medical records. The back cover of this brochure contains a wallet size card that you can complete and carry with you to tell others that you have an advance directive.

Can I be required to sign an advance directive?

No. An advance directive is not required for admission to a hospital, nursing home, or other health care facility. You cannot be refused admission to a hospital, nursing home, or other health care facility because you do not have an advance directive.

Can I be required to complete an advance directive as a condition of my insurance coverage?

No. You cannot be required to complete an advance directive as a condition for obtaining a life or health insurance policy. Also, having, or not having, an advance directive has no effect on your current health or life insurance coverage, or health benefits.

Can I use my advance directive to make an organ donation upon my death?

Yes. The sample combined directive and instruction directive included with this brochure provide a place for you to state your wishes regarding organ donation. Also, on the inside back cover of this brochure is a wallet size organ donor card. If you decide to make a gift of your organs upon your death please complete the card and carry it with you at all times. For further information regarding organ donation you should contact either an organ procurement agency or your local hospital.

Will another state honor my advance directive?

It is likely that your advance directive will be honored in another state, but this is not guaranteed.

What if I already have a living will?

While you may want to review your existing living will or advance directive and make sure it reflects your wishes, there is no legal requirement that you do so.

POSTSCRIPT

She is still alive.

It seems that part, if not all, of my wife's medical problems may be hysteria (or mimicing). Not too long ago, she was written about in a leading medical journal as a classical hysteric for that disease entity. Her (now) attending neurologist told me this. He further said that her diagnosis (of Huntington's Disease) was based on her outward presenting symptoms, not on MRI or CAT scans, which showed no clear cell death or black striations of the brain, which is usually (always?) the case.

I only mention this because it would be most strange to let a woman, of anyone else, die or *agree to die* because of a mental problem (hysteria), not a physical one.

In more broad terms, should prople with psychosomatic illnesses in general, who want to be sick or die, be allowed to?

Interesting question, isn't it? Does a person have the freedom to keep their state of mind, however odd is might seem to others?

Even more broadly, should there be some kind of psychological relativism where each person be allowed to live in whatever psychological or psycho-biological state they want? Another interesting question, both psychiatrically and socially.

* * *

On March 24, 1993, an article appeared on the first page of *The New York Times* announcing that the defective gene causing Huntington's Disease had been found. Although the article stated some experts felt it might be a few years before this could be translated into a cure, people with the disease had new hope. It seems then that much of the anguish about making a life or death decision for my wife had become *moot*. If it is so that this discovery, along with new drugs which may reverse the course of the disease, then my wife may live longer than myself. The living wills which had been signed by patients allowing for the use of life support systems were probably a good thing. Some of those that had signed a living will disallowing life support had died already.

These facts, of course, raise a more general question involving many diseases, whether signing off from life support systems is a wise move, since in some cases a cure will be found years later.

In any case, the news was well received by the 25,000 people who have the disease in the U.S.A. and the 125,000 who were at risk.

Genetic medicine had come into its own and may allow people to live 140 years, as we have said. Again science will produce solutions to many medical problems. But again, the solutions will generate, possibly, the problem of supporting the half of the population who will be over 65. Yes, new moral decisions will have to be made.

Nevertheless, it goes without saying that we as a family are ecstatic over the probable cure for Huntington's Disease.

Eternal Life

About the same time as the discovery of the Huntington's gene, it was widely reported in scientific journals and other publications that three genes determined whether any cell would live or die. The evidence suggested that theoretically a person could have eternal life.

I asked my students whether they would like man-made eternal life. None of them wanted it. I asked them why, and they generally did not know why, other than that they had the false impression that they would be old and shriveled up. They did raise questions about how society could handle such a thing.

I said, "It would certainly be a problem."

Later, I mused to myself. In this book and in this relatively short length of time, I have passed through the Hell of genetic disease into the Purgatory of knowing that Huntington's Disease could be cured and maybe reversed, now to the somewhat dubious Heaven of eternal life, through the miracles of genetic engineering, that few people seem to want. As a student said, "Eternity is a long time, and I would probably get bored after several thousand years."

"How odd," I said to myself, "From Hell to Heaven in a decade or two." It's been an interesting trip, sort of like reading *The Divine Comedy* by Dante and falling asleep periodically while in *The Inferno*, waking up to read *Purgatorio* and contemplating the man-made *Paradiso*.

INDEX

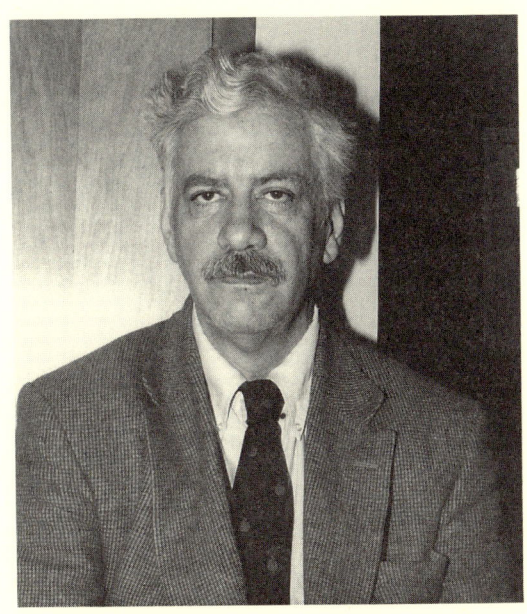

NOTES ON AUTHOR

Dr. James Hill Parker is a professor of Sociology and Anthropology at Long Island University in Brooklyn, N.Y. He teaches in the fields of medical sociology, the sociology of mental illness and socio-biology.

He has published 40 articles, some in the area of medical sociology in a variety of professional journals and The New York Times. He has also conducted a two-city study on the Community Participation of Health Professionals and Businessmen.

His previous four books have all dealt with social systems and the possible breakdown of such systems.

This book is a continuation of this approach and a lifetime interest in medical sociology.